Praise for
The Power of the Hollow Bone

"I am confident that this book will support and help many people. It has been said that the healing teachings will arise all over the planet in different forms, and in different ways and this is one that will open the hearts and the healing power of many."

—David T. Kyle,
author of *Energy Teachings of The Three*

"In *The Power of the Hollow Bone* Phoenix Rising Star offers holistic healers an accessible overview of timeless truths of healing that make all the difference in the outcomes of our clients. If you are sometimes puzzled by how to help people with complex, challenging issues, read this treasure of a book."

—Darren Starwynn, OMD,
author of *Awakening the Avatar Within*

"Phoenix has written an enlightening, must-read guide to becoming a hollow bone or conduit for the Divine Source. It is a simple way to clear away anything that could possibly clog the bone of our spirit and mind. When we can move our ego and rational mind out of the way to channel the Divine power of the universe through us, anything is possible."

—Michael Drake,
author of *The Shamanic Drum*

"A beautifully well-written book that is easily understood and relatable. *The Power of The Hollow Bone* helps you have a greater impact with your clients regardless of whether you are new to the holistic healing practices or well-established. This is a must-read for deep results that come quickly with ease and grace that is always for the highest and best."

—Florence Buie,
artist and holistic practitioner, Where Art Meets Healing LLC

"The Power of the Hollow Bone offers sequential, easy-to-follow steps, and is easily applied to your holistic healing practice. The easy-to-read style with case studies and supplementary material makes this a captivating practitioners' manual, filling me with hope for healing humanity and peace on Earth."

—Russell Sutton,
holistic practitioner and director of Love Energy Healing

"Used as a stand-alone or an add-on to an existing practice, being the hollow bone is the way to be the conduit for Source and see transformative results. "

—Katrina K. Abeyta,
holistic healing practitioner

The
POWER
of the
HOLLOW
BONE

The
POWER
of the
HOLLOW
BONE

**SERVE MORE CLIENTS, SEE FAST TRANSFORMATIONAL
HEALING, AND MAKE A BIGGER IMPACT WITH YOUR
HOLISTIC WELLNESS BUSINESS**

PHOENIX RISING STAR

Disclaimer:
This book is for informational and educational purposes only. The information and education provided is not intended or implied to supplement or replace professional medical treatment, advice, and/or diagnosis. Please consult a physician or health care provider if you have any health concerns.

Neither Personal Energy Transformation LLC or the author offer any representations, guarantees, or warranties, of any variety, regarding the book in any way including, but not limited to, effectiveness, safety, harm, or results achieved as a result of your use of the book. The book is offered **"AS IS"** and without representations, guarantees, or warranties of any kind, including but not limited to, implied warranties of merchantability and fitness for a particular purpose, neither express nor implied, to the extent permitted by law. Neither Personal Energy Transformation, LLC or the author are liable for damages of any kind related to your use of the book or any information contained or discussed therein.

Editor: Lydia Reineck, LinkedIn.com/in/lydia-reineck-277329b
Production & Publishing Consultant: AuthorPreneur Publishing Inc.—authorpreneurbooks.com
Cover Designer: Zizi Iryaspraha Subiyarta
Interior Designer: Amit Dey—amitdey2528@gmail.com

ISBN: 979-8-9886826-0-8 (paperback)
ISBN: 979-8-9886826-1-5 (eBook)
ISBN: 979-8-9886826-2-2 (audiobook)

HEA032000 HEALTH & FITNESS / Alternative Therapies
OCC011010 BODY, MIND & SPIRIT / Healing / Energy

Contents

Overview

This manual is for you if you are looking for additional ways to help others on their healing path, whether they're family and friends or paying clients.

This manual is for you if you are seeking faster and better results in your holistic practice without working harder.

This manual is for you if you are ready to make a bigger impact on the world as a healing practitioner and don't know how.

And this manual is for you if you are ready to up-level your life and your holistic practice and make your unbelievable . . . believable.

This book has four parts:

Part One: My Backwards Story

Part Two: Finding the Origin of the Hollow Bone of Healing

Part Three: Putting it All Together in Your Holistic Practice

Part Four: How to Be the Hollow Bone on a Daily Basis—And Why

Each section details the necessary steps involved in being the hollow bone for others and helps you understand how you can do this. In Part One: My Backwards Story, I share how I had to work backwards from that first experience with Archangel

Michael and figure out how I could replicate being the hollow bone. I detail the steps I've learned that are essential, and I share case studies of my students. I also include guided meditations to help you experience the necessary steps so you can see better and faster results in your practice—without working harder.

Finding the Origin of the Hollow Bone of Healing in Part Two came as a divine intervention. After seeking it for three years, I "stumbled" upon an obscure reference that led me to deeply understand the traditional ways of healing but from a shamanic perspective. I learned about levels of consciousness and how to access ancient ways and knowledge. I've also included some of the shamanic journeys my students themselves have experienced through accessing the traditional, ancient ways of healing.

Part Three: Putting it All Together in Your Holistic Practice helps you apply being the hollow bone to your existing practice, using everything you've just learned, whether you are the hollow bone as an add-on or a stand-alone. I have included case studies, extra training, and a checklist to assist you in being the hollow bone in your practice.

Part Four: How to BE the Hollow Bone on a Daily Basis answers the question: where do we go from here? Because it's not enough to just use this in your practice. Being the hollow bone becomes a way of living, a way of seeing with the eyes of the Divine (or Source), of speaking with the words of the Divine or Source. When you live this way, miracles and messages are a common occurrence for you and for everyone around you. This transformation for you happens and you begin to witness more client transformation with faster results.

**This is how you begin to make a
bigger impact on the world:
This is the way of the shaman,
This is the way of the healer,
This is the path of ascension.**

This is the way home.

Important information: *Access all your included free
meditations, journeys, and training materials in one place!*

**Register for your FREE Hollow Bone
Audios, Videos, Checklists
Supplement Materials**
https://www.ask-the-angels.org/offers/vLUgb9ny

**Already registered?
Access your account here**
https://www.ask-the-angels.org/login

Introduction

I 'll never forget seeing Archangel Michael with my inner eyesight. He was tall and wore armor and flowing purple robes. His light brown hair was long and slightly curly. Incredibly handsome. I had never "seen" him before. Usually I'm auditory and hear him talking. But to see him like this stunned me. I felt frozen, not with fear, but with the love emanating from him. All I could do was observe as he reached into the spine of my client, as she laid on a massage table. He pulled out something that looked like ticker tape, or a wide ribbon.

Pulling it up and away from her body, he placed his thumb on one side of the ribbon and his forefinger pressed on the other side. Starting at the top of the ribbon, closest to her head, his hand and fingers slid slowly down the ribbon to the base of her spine and continued to slide back and forth, up and down on the ribbon. Turning to me, he smiled and said, "There! Now that we're clearing off all the ancestral cellular memory she's been carrying, she'll have a much easier time manifesting exactly what she wants. She'll be very happy with the results!"

Then, having completed his "clearing," he tucked the ribbon back into her spine, turned to me, bowed and left the room. I sat still in amazement and awe—still feeling frozen, still feeling the love and knowing intuitively that something really profound had just happened—but not being able to make sense of it.

My client had slept deeply the entire time and was unaware of his presence. When she awakened, her eyes opened wide. She appeared relaxed as though she'd had a great deep sleep. And she wanted to know what happened. I explained that the angels had cleared her ancestral memory, which would help her manifest better. She swung her legs off the table, filled with energy and promised to keep me posted on her progress.

After she left, I sat in meditation and asked the angels I usually talk with, "What just happened?"

"Why, that was the hollow bone of healing!"

I took my time responding, and then said, "Well, that wasn't my normal M.O. (method of operating) I use for healing sessions."

Their answer? "No, it hasn't been. But it is now."

That was the beginning of my backwards story, because I knew this was powerful. I knew what I'd just experienced, and it was up to me to figure out how to replicate being the "hollow bone of healing" so everyone could do it and see transformative results like I ultimately did.

Only I had no idea just how life-changing being the hollow bone of healing really could be. That was more than three years ago, and I've learned so much since that time!

When I first became aware of being the hollow bone of healing, I sat down and quickly wrote my previous book, *The Hollow Bone of Healing: Miracles and Messages from the Quantum Field of Source Energy*. This self-healing manual for beginners was meant as a series of steps to assist individuals in becoming a higher version of themselves. As a foundational book it provides the basics to get started with the hollow bone of healing for yourself. There are free guided meditations to better assist each step.

Now, more than three years later, having taught the process to hundreds of students and learned so much, I'm able to share deeper knowledge and wisdom about being the hollow bone of healing and how it up-levels your holistic practice and your life.

Being the hollow bone of healing is a process. It isn't a technique, it's a level of consciousness. And as you tap into it with your intention and awareness, your intuition heightens, your connection to the Divine or Source Energy becomes stronger, and your ability to safely access higher realms of helpers improves your skill in being the pipeline or channel for the miracles of Source Energy.

There are no limits to this work. No "invisible ceilings" to this process. Nothing that says, "oh, it only works in this way, but not in other ways." No "you have to use these hand positions only." Or "everyone gets the same treatment regardless of their presenting issue." The hollow bone of healing is the pipeline to the Divine, to Source Energy. Source never runs out of ideas or ways to help, and the results are always for the highest and best, no matter what that is.

Once you have learned how to be the hollow bone for yourself, some of you will want to be able to do this with and for others.

If you are ready for this, read on!

PART ONE

My Backwards
Story

CHAPTER 1

What You Can Expect

After that experience with Archangel Michael when I was told that being the hollow bone of healing was my new M.O., I knew I had to figure out how it happened. I had to trace backwards to the very first step that initiated this and go from there so I could better help others to step into being the hollow bone of healing.

I thought about how our session began. My client came in with a laundry list of how she wanted her life to be different. It was pretty convoluted, actually. Her list began with her relationship, which was rocky. It continued with her finances, which were in short supply. Next, her career wasn't exactly how she wanted it, but she was afraid to do something different or look for something better. And last, she was beginning to have some health issues that may or may not have been induced from stress.

Whew! I didn't even know how to begin helping her. I had been working as an intuitive healer, where I sat in silence and received my guidance for what to "do". So, it didn't bother me that I didn't know what to do. I figured Source Energy would tell me.

Opening the Heart

But first, because she was fairly agitated, I led us both in a guided meditation to calm her down and help both of us open our hearts. Once she was in a good place, she laid on the massage table and waited for me.

Now, doing a guided meditation to open our hearts was not new to me. I'd done that before with previous clients. But I'd never had the kind of results I had with seeing Archangel Michael. So, I knew that heart-opening guided meditation, as important as it was, was not everything. There had to be more to the process of being the hollow bone of healing than just this meditation.

When I first wrote the book *The Hollow Bone of Healing*, I knew the heart-opening meditation was important. But I had no idea just how profound it could be. I will share with you how I learned to offer the heart-opening meditation differently, and how I maximized results of the client with this meditation.

Your Safety Net

Next, I remember what I said silently as I waited to receive my guidance. I said jokingly, "Okay, we're going to have to bring in the big guns for this one, as I really don't know what to do here." What I meant, of course, was "please bring in the highest and best helpers for support." That could include any spiritual helpers in the higher consciousness category, helpers such as angels, archangels, ascended masters, spirits of light, spirits of love, spirits of compassion, and so on. I wasn't asking for Archangel Michael specifically. I just asked for his category of helpers, and since he was apparently the highest and best for this particular job, he came in to assist.

Since then, the angels have explained to me that when asking for the highest and best spiritual helpers, you will only have helpers that are for your highest and best. No other energies or levels of consciousness are allowed, which means you have just created your safety net. No more opening to any and all helpers because our 3-D world has a lot of different energies out there. We don't have time to play with them all. We want only the highest and best helpers because that request brings us the best and fastest help and support.

Included in Part 2 are case studies with my students and their experiences with highest and best helpers. Learn how asking for the highest and best assists you in safely being the hollow bone of healing.

Allowing

After calling in the big guns, I sat in meditation with an open heart and allowed Source Energy to guide me. Or in this case, I waited for the spiritual helpers to appear. When I saw Archangel Michael, I remember feeling frozen, in a field of love, unable to move or do anything other than to observe. This perception is what I now call allowing—allowing our highest-level spiritual helpers to come in and do what they do best. We are in a place of being and receiving; we are passive, not directing or doing. Coming from a place of trust, we are trusting in Source, and we are trusting ourselves to recognize and believe that what we are experiencing is not from us. It is from beyond us. Source has an intelligence of its own that goes far beyond our own, always knowing exactly what it's doing. And it's always perfect.

Read more about allowing and find out how you can get out of your head and learn to think with your heart so you can be a better hollow bone of healing.

Detaching from the Outcome

Since I had no idea how to help my client, this particular case was easy for me to detach from the outcome. Whatever happened would be for her highest and best, no matter how that presented itself. *Enough said!*

But sometimes detaching is not so easy, especially when, as holistic practitioners, we have a deep yearning to be of service, to help people, to heal people, to make things right. Sometimes we get in the way without meaning to.

> Learn what happens when we get in the way
> and why detaching is so important when being
> the hollow bone of healing.

Receiving Permission

Obviously if you're working with a client, you probably have permission to be the hollow bone of healing. And if you're working with a family member, you probably have permission also. But what about someone who you think "obviously needs healing"? Can you just be the hollow bone?

> Read what the angels told me about the role of permission
> and how you can see better and faster results from clients
> when you exercise the role of permission.

The Roles of Healing

Many times, we hear the word healing and we think physical healing. A tumor disappears, an eye infection gets better, the stomach distress is improved. But healing is so much more than physical healing.

Learn how healing can present itself,
so you can help clients experience better and
faster results and recognize them
when they happen!

Ready to find out more? Let's get started!

CHAPTER 2

Opening the Heart

Initially, I led my client in a heart-opening guided meditation to calm her down and help both of us open our hearts. Once she was in a good place, she laid on the massage table and waited for me.

When I first wrote the book *The Hollow Bone of Healing*, I knew the heart-opening meditation was important. But I had no idea just how profound it could be. I've heard from so many people who have said how healing that meditation is—how peaceful, serene. It puts them in the place of everything and the place of nothing. This is probably the most important meditation when being the hollow bone of healing! The heart meditation has become the foundation for everything we do.

But I had a few things to figure out first. First—yes, I heard from so many people who were having wonderful results with this meditation. Yet I also heard from people who were having difficulty with it.

"I have a hard time getting into my heart."

"I don't even know what unconditional love is! Maybe I have it with my dog, but
I'm not even sure about him!"

"I can't seem to get this meditation."

And so on.

What I learned from that is how much pain we carry in our hearts. When we have heart hurt, we tend to close off our hearts from ever hurting again, ever loving again—because we don't want to feel that pain. If we have multiple heart hurts, we close off all feeling, out of fear that everything hurts.

When we're closed off in our hearts, it's darn hard to decide one day to trust and open up to a guided meditation where you might lose control, and then, who knows what will happen! So, we hold on even tighter to our pain.

The problem with this is that the harder we hold on, the less love we can remember or take in. The less love we take in, the harder it is to heal. So, holding on really creates a challenging situation where fear of pain or hurt is in control and love has no place. So, I had to come at this meditation from several angles.

First, I started by taking more time with it. I made this a much longer meditation. I talk more slowly. I pause more. I give more time for silence. This slower, longer pace seems to have helped a lot of people. It gives them time to settle in, especially if their brain wants to control the meditation and make it safe.

Next, I began with a place in nature, because everyone has some place in nature that they love and feel good about. Everyone can relate to nature, even if it's a park. I really hone in on the details of the rich beauty that exists in nature, helping people to zero in on the specific colors of their specific place, especially the colors of green, which is nature's healing color, and blue, which is the color of the angels. Also, we listen to the sounds that are specific to that place—the water, wind, animals, birds, or the hush of profound silence. I encourage them to get in touch with the feeling of the sun on their skin, knowing it's perfect. I encourage them to note the unique fragrances of flowers, soil, water, and air, to observe animals and birds and flowers, to really be present in nature so that they allow nature to open their hearts, little by little.

And that works really well for many people. They're not as anxious about trying to feel unconditional love because they're more relaxed in a non-threatening environment. They now have an easier time with this meditation.

Still, I found that after a year or so, they needed something newer, even though students now were doing the longer meditation and really grounding into nature. They seemed to need something different that still opened their hearts. That's when I created a new meditation with The Spirits of Love and Light to bring them into their hearts, allowing us all to really see through the eyes of Love and Light. My students love this new meditation.

Now, that time when I witnessed Archangel Michael with my client, I was used to offering a guided meditation to open our hearts. However, up to that point, I'd never had the kind of results I had that day with Archangel Michael. So, I then knew that the heart-opening guided meditation, as important as it was, was not everything. There had to be more to this process of being the hollow bone of healing than just this meditation.

Experience both heart-opening guided
meditations in The Power of the Hollow
Bone Supplement Materials.

**Register for your FREE Hollow Bone
Audios, Videos, Checklists
Supplement Materials**
https://www.ask-the-angels.org/offers/vLUgb9ny

**Already registered?
Access your account here**
https://www.ask-the-angels.org/login

Read on to find what I discovered about
Your Safety Net and how important it is
to have during a session.

CHAPTER 3

Your Safety Net

I think many times when we are first learning how to access energy and offer healing, we get so thrilled being able to do this that we just invite in every helper who's out there! While that can be exciting, it can also be scary. After all, in our 3-D world we have all kinds of energies out there, and not all of them are kind, loving, and considerate. Just walking into the supermarket, if you're sensitive, you can feel different energies from different people. Anger from some. Sorrow from others. Indifference from many. Exhaustion on most faces. So, ask yourself, is that the kind of energy you want to access for healing?

No, of course not. And you might say, "yes, but that's not the kind of energy I'm going to find in a healing session!" Or is it?

When working with energy, it's really important to have safe boundaries, boundaries that prevent unwanted energies from interfering. Calling in your favorite helpers, such as Archangel Michael or Angel Metatron or others, is certainly a great place to begin. Angels, archangels, ascended masters are all high in vibrational energy, and pure. You'll receive high and pure healing with them. But what if there was a spiritual helper who was even better for the healing session, and you didn't know that or even know who it might be? How can you include them?

When I asked for the "big guns" in my client session and I saw Archangel Michael, I believed I was asking for those helpers who were for my client's highest and best. I didn't know it was going to be Archangel Michael. I didn't know Archangel Michael could change ancestral patterns by cleaning off the DNA in the spine. I simply couldn't fathom it because I'd never experienced it before. So, I didn't know to ask for him.

When we ask for the highest and best, we always get it.

And here's why this becomes your safety net.

When you ask for the highest and best, that's what shows up. AND, the only result these helpers deliver is whatever is for the client's highest and best—no matter what that is. PLUS, no other spiritual helpers can come in if they're not for the highest and best.

That limits the playing ground for the chaotic 3-D energies that are unwanted. Because we've asked for the highest and best, anything that's not from those categories simply can't play with us.

I've included some examples of being the hollow bone of healing and experiencing what happens when you ask for the highest and best spiritual helpers on behalf of the client. These examples are from students and practitioners of The Healing Angel Protocol™, but as you'll find out later in the book, you can be the hollow bone of healing as part of any holistic practice.

From Marie Forest, Healing Angel Protocol™ Practitioner and Team Leader in training:

"The person had had COVID that went into pneumonia, and we were trying to heal that. I was focusing on the heart chakra (of my client). The angels came in and there was this little mushroom on the heart. They screwed off the cap of the mushroom, and then started pulling out all these little threads of stuff that looked like filament from a camera film or something, but the threads were covered in this green slime. I was pulling green slime from the threads I could see. These particles were so long, they were extending into the lungs. The angels and I were pulling them out the heart, and the angels just took the particles away. They put the cap back on the mushroom, and then we finished the healing session. Next time, they came back to the heart. They took the cap off again and put the filaments back in, but this time, the filaments were all shining and glowing, just beautifully brilliant. And they each were stamped with a healing code. The angels said they were putting this healing code into the heart center to finish releasing the virus from the body. The green slime was the residual of the virus that they cleaned off. It was like, "wow, okay. I just got to watch the whole thing!" She felt so much better immediately!"

From Karen Sayago, Healing Angel Protocol™ Practitioner

"I worked with a client who wanted to eliminate physical injuries and create a state of greater health and wellness. He also wanted to reclaim his sovereignty.

"Archangel Michael came in and gave him the Sword of Truth. It was placed in my client's hands, so that the point was straight up. It wasn't heavy. It was light energy. Archangel Michael told him he needed to be filled with the Truth and Trust.

"The Spirit of Truth and the Spirit of Trust also came in. The Trust energy expanded and expanded in the energy field as Archangel Michael's sword was held.

"Archangel Gabriel also came in to move out stale energy. Gabriel was helping the inner sight /intuition/ third eye to clear and open and also clearing thoughts in the brain that held old beliefs. All cells through the body from feet to neck and brain were worked on to heal old cellular memory. I was told the cells would regenerate into their healthiest, purest essence of themselves.

"The client was seeing the healing as it was being done and thinking I was seeing the same thing, but I was visualizing it in a different way. He was very excited about what he witnessed and felt healing immediately."

From Donna Wolf, Healing Angel Protocol™ Practitioner

"I worked with a client who was feeling ungrounded and rather fragile and nervous. During the session Yeshua [Jesus] came in with nomadic monks to offer strong protection. There was a lot of clearing of restless 'unbelonging' energy from his field. His guides worked with his Root Chakra the entire time. Old hobo shoes and old moccasins were removed. Old cloaks of consciousness were removed. He was aligned with Cellular Memories of Wisdom gained through deeply challenging lifetimes that prepared him to serve as a teacher and mentor of Nourishing Self-Care. His inner voice expressed awe as he indeed felt 'I Am Loved! I Can Love! I Feel Love!' His inner eyes were also cleared of veils in relation to feeling safe, being 'rooted' as an Embodied Soul—seeing the Blessings of What Has Been and What Is so he can embrace 'Being Here Now.' On impulse from Guides, I was prompted to kiss his feet as a symbolic expression that he was partnered with their Presence.

"After the session, he went from fragile to calm and strong."

From Marisa Martucci, Healing Angel Protocol™ Practitioner and Team Leader

"I went to the doctor with some pain in my ovaries. He said it appeared that there was a cyst there but needed to confirm with more tests, and then he'd know what kind of treatment would be necessary, whether surgery or something else. As I was headed for my appointment, I called in whoever was for my highest and best and asked for healing. I saw Angel Ariel's face and felt a very comforting presence. Then, while I was in the waiting room, I felt her come in again. Again, I saw her face and felt her comforting presence. But then I felt like she reached inside me and removed something. I had no idea what it was. They finally called my name for my tests. During my tests, they took pictures and conferred. They called in additional people. Took more tests and conferred. I was getting nervous about what was going on.

"Finally, they said, 'Ok. You can go home now.'

"I said, 'What? What is happening?'

"They said, 'Well, we could tell something had been there. But now there's nothing. You can go home now.'"

Not all our spiritual helpers are angels or archangels. Karen witnessed the Spirits of Truth and Trust, which are high consciousness forms. Donna experienced Yeshua, or Jesus, who is considered to be an Ascended Master. We never know who our highest and best will be, but when we open to them, we always receive our highest and best.

While asking for the highest and best is important, allowing ourselves and our clients to receive that highest and best takes healing to the next level. It takes being the hollow bone of healing to the next level.

> Read on to learn how to think with your
> heart and always allow.

CHAPTER 4

Allowing

When we ask for our highest-level spiritual helpers to come in and do what they do best, we are, in fact, passive—in a place of being and receiving, not directing or doing. Coming from a place of trust, we are trusting in Source, and we are trusting ourselves to recognize and believe that what we are experiencing is not from us. It is from beyond us. Source has an intelligence of its own and knows exactly what it's doing. And it's always perfect.

The problem is that as holistic healers, or in a holistic practice, we've had training to rely on. Sometimes we have lots of modalities because we are life-long learners and love learning more and more. Sometimes our calling has demanded that in order to be a certain kind of practitioner, we have levels of training, years of training, or even repeat training in order to maintain our certification. And sometimes we've told ourselves we just needed a lot of tools in our toolbox in order to better serve.

There's nothing wrong with any of this—until it gets in the way.

Being the hollow bone of healing is not the same as being intuitive. It's taking your intuition and your training to a deeper level of being, namely, where the Divine or Source Energy does all the work, and your only job is to be the "hollow bone" for the Divine or Source to come through. This is how miracles happen.

It's not about how hard we're working, or how much we know. It's about how well we are able to let go of our ego, open our hearts, and allow Source to come through love.

And there we are again: back with the first theme of love!

But it's true. Love is what comes through when we're the hollow bone of healing. That's the only thing that heals. And the Divine or Source Energy is the source of all love and therefore the source for all healing.

We are not doing the work when we are the hollow bone of healing.

We are receiving and allowing the Divine or Source Energy to do what it does best: healing with love.

The biggest challenge for holistic practitioners is to get out of the way. To stop trying to look at a client and think, "Hmm. What do I have in my toolbox that would help this person?"

Not that there's anything wrong with that. But it's a different level of consciousness than having the Divine or Source Energy do the work. Think about asking yourself, who would I like to receive healing from? A trainer or Source?

Don't get me wrong. I was an intuitive healer for two decades. I loved it. I loved sitting and receiving guidance and being told what to do. And that worked. Until it didn't.

When it stopped working was when I saw Archangel Michael perform miracles I didn't know how to do, or even fathom that they were possible.

That's when the angels said to me, "It hasn't been your M.O. (method of operating) but it is now." Meaning, that once you step into this way of being, there is no going back.

Why would you?

Why not continue to see miracles, healing, and guidance that is so much better than anything you could offer, even with all your training? Why would you want to do anything else? It's less effort on your part with greater results. The payoffs are tremendous. You get happier, more satisfied clients that turn into repeat customers for life. It's a win-win for everyone just by being the hollow bone of healing and allowing.

This is the first step to getting out of your head and thinking with your heart—remembering that the results have nothing to do with you. You are not responsible for the outcome. Source has your back. Source has everyone's back. And the results are amazing. Every time.

The second step of getting out of your head and thinking with your heart is to do the heart-opening meditation before your client walks in the door. So, when you open your eyes, you are seeing your client with the eyes of love. You are touching with your eyes. Your heart is wide open to Source Energy. You are allowing Source to work through you. *It is enough!*

The third step is to keep reminding yourself of Step #1 and repeating Step #2 as often as necessary.

Now that I have talked about how the results are amazing and perfect every time, there is a caveat to that. Sometimes we have a preconceived notion of what "perfect" results should be, and what we witness doesn't match up to that. The perfect results may not appear as we "think" they should. ***YOU WILL GET THIS!*** It's a process. And it's a process that can be learned. You will never regret it.

Want to listen to the heart-opening meditation again?

**Register for your FREE Hollow Bone
Audios, Videos, Checklists
Supplement Materials**
https://www.ask-the-angels.org/offers/vLUgb9ny

**Already registered?
Access your account here**
https://www.ask-the-angels.org/login

Read on to find out how important it is to detach from
the outcome and how that allows you to be
a better "hollow bone."

CHAPTER 5

Detaching from the Outcome

I was working with a suicidal client who lived in another state. We were on the phone, and she was saying things like, "I should just end it all. I can't go on like this." Of course, her comments were making me increasingly nervous that she might try to commit suicide.

She even had a plan. "I'll just take a bunch of pills and never wake up."

I was on the phone for quite a while, offering lots of love. Finally, I got her to agree she wouldn't take action for at least 24 hours, and that the next day she would either call me or text me. I asked her if she'd like to receive a session in the meantime, and she agreed.

I was in a pretty wired state and needed to move around. So, I decided I could walk outside and send a session at the same time. I was at the point where it really didn't matter if I sat still in meditation or was more active, as I knew Source Energy was doing all the work.

I began to walk on my favorite walk that was partly in neighborhoods, and partly in the forest. As I walked, I was praying, "Please don't let her commit suicide. Please don't let her commit suicide. Please don't let her commit suicide."

And nothing was happening.

No energy was flowing through me.

No sign of Source Energy.

No feeling. No awareness of spiritual helpers. Nothing.

Finally, I literally stopped on my walk and asked internally, "What is going on?"

Immediately I heard, "You are trying to push the agenda."

I got it immediately. I was putting my idea of the outcome of the session into the healing session. Of course, that's not how it works. Being the hollow bone of healing means Source Energy is doing the work. I have no say in the outcome. The results are always perfect even if they aren't what I thought they should be. I resolved to talk to the angels later about that as I still had some questions. But even then, I knew enough to get out of my own way.

So, I went back to my heart, asked for the highest and best on behalf of my client, no matter what that was, and allowed.

Boom! It was like a switch turned on. All this energy flowed through me powerfully. I knew something was happening, but I had no idea what it was. It flowed and flowed as I walked. When it was complete, the feeling diminished, and I knew the session was done.

When I got home, I sat in meditation to ask the angels why it was "wrong" to ask that my client not commit suicide. Here's what I heard.

"It's not wrong to ask for anything. But the problem was that you were asking to be the hollow bone for her healing. And that means you had to detach from the outcome, no matter what that was. It is not up to you to judge her actions as bad or good. It's up to you to be the cleanest, clearest bone you can be so we can help her. We do not judge anyone if they decide they've had enough of the 3-D life. When they're done, they'll find a way to leave. And who are you to decide someone should stay longer and suffer more?" This was not said to me in judgment. It was said as a kind, benevolent grandfather would to a small child who didn't understand. And I hadn't understood, so I was grateful for this extra knowledge and wisdom and the remembrance to not judge. Grateful to go farther with my training in being the hollow bone.

This was a very powerful lesson that sometimes is challenging to do! But when I felt all that energy flow to her, even though I didn't know what was happening, I knew something was happening—much more than when I was trying direct the session.

And I have to admit, I was very happy to receive her call the next day saying she felt better.

I'm not saying it's easy to detach from the outcome. I've had many clients who are in great pain, great sorrow, great distress, great trauma, and they just want it to be gone. What I have learned is when we "hold on" tightly, asking for what we desire fervently doesn't bring it to us faster. In fact, "holding on" can keep it away because we're not letting the Divine or Source energy in. We're actually preventing any help and support because of our focus on one condition or one result. When asking for the highest and best, the result may not be healing or curing. The highest and best result may be empowerment, or learning the lesson of compassion, or learning how to receive, or something entirely different. We simply don't know what our soul came here to learn until we're in the middle of it. Even then, it may not be clear to us.

Here's a beautiful example of how asking for the highest and detaching from the outcome brings greater results than what my client was hoping for.

My client was experiencing lots of health challenges. Because her doctors were puzzled, all they did was offer her more meds. In desperation, she asked me for a healing session.

Following up the next day, I asked her how she was doing?

"You're going to be upset!" she said.

"I'm not going to be upset," I said. "It's your session!"

"Well, I'm not better!"

"What are you, then?" I asked.

"I think the problem is all the meds I'm on. I think I need to sit down with my doctor and figure out exactly what I need and what I don't."

Now *that* was clearly her highest and best coming through.

Why? Because she became her best health advocate, no longer relying on someone telling her what was good for her but now taking charge of her life and her health. Something she hadn't been doing. If all her symptoms had magically healed from the session, what would she have gained from that? Sure, she might have felt better. But what about the next time she was sick? Then what?

With this outcome of empowerment, she was now able to take charge of her healing, no matter what kind of healer she works with. She's now empowered to sit down and be an active part of her healing plan.

Lesson learned: ***Always allow for the something better.***

Detach from **what you *think* you need**.

You will *always* receive the something better. Even if it's **not what you *thought*.**

CHAPTER 6

The Role of Permission

In the previous section, I was working with regular clients, yet, with the suicidal client, when it came time to offer a session, I still asked for permission.

Why? Because the angels have told me over and over again, "Don't assume."

"Don't assume that because you see someone you 'think' needs healing that they do. You might see someone walking on crutches with only one leg and in obvious pain, and think, well, doesn't that person need healing? Our answer is, that depends. Maybe. Maybe not. Sure, we don't like to see suffering either. But what if that person needed that pain and that experience in order to learn what their soul wanted them to learn when they came here? What if those experiences were the best ways to learn those lessons, whatever they might be? What if by offering healing, you were actually interfering with the learning of those lessons? Creating a lessening of the pain or a changing of the perspective that created more dependency than independency. From that perspective, we don't feel that healing would be for the highest and best. And we ask that you always ask for permission to offer it, and not assume anything."

I understood the transmission. And I understood it when I had a student ask me, "Well, how is it such a bad thing to offer love?"

My answer came from the angels. "Offering love is never a bad thing. But directing healing because you believe it's necessary is like pushing your own agenda. You are trying to direct the outcome. You are not being the hollow bone of healing. You are doing your thing. This is the awareness we want to bring to what you are doing. It's better to ask first and be the hollow bone and detach from the outcome of what that is, than to try to push the water and direct the outcome yourself."

Shortly after this transmission, I was working with a client who had backed herself into a corner energetically, meaning, she was hurting inside but afraid to acknowledge it. She was depressed and lethargic and not doing much to change that. She asked me for help, but wanted astrology, which I don't do. She was avoiding anything that would help her to confront the emotional cause.

I figured that since we'd worked together before, it wouldn't hurt to send her a quick session. After all, I'd had permission before to work with her, so what would be the harm?

Well, nothing happened. By that I mean I felt nothing. No energy flowed through me to her. Nothing happened. It was like a giant hand with the palm facing me with the word STOP! So, I waited a moment, and then asked the angels what was going on.

Here was their reply: "You are not receiving permission at this time, even though in the past you have been given permission. Right now, she needs to figure this out for herself, and not have someone 'rescue' her. It's really okay for her to be in this dark place. It is the catalyst she needs to bring in the light."

I got it. I shouldn't push *my* agenda and assume healing would be helpful. Even when I think I'm being helpful, if I don't have permission, nothing will flow through me. Being the hollow bone has nothing to do with me. It has everything to do with the Divine or Source.

In this case, the Divine or Source was not giving permission, as opposed to the actual client. Be open to the highest and best, ask permission, and listen with your heart.

Find out more about the role of healing in the next section, and all the ways healing can be experienced. This will help you be a better hollow bone and help clients who are receiving both expected and unexpected results.

CHAPTER 7

What is Healing?

So many times, we think it's obvious. A person gets sick. Then they heal and get better. But what does that mean? Is it always physical?

What are all the ways we heal?

Healing is defined in these ways, according to thefreedictionary.com

1. to make healthy, whole, or sound: restore to health; free from ailment.

2. to repair or reconcile; settle: to heal the rift between them.

3. to free from evil; cleanse; purify: to heal the soul.

The phrases "free from ailment, healing the rift, heal the soul" all indicate that healing is not all physical. I remember a time when I had a client who walked into my office with difficulty. He was stooped, using a walker, and had lines in his face, aging him. He came in with his wife, who appeared to be very youthful and slim. Moving easily and well, and yet with an underlying stress and tension.

Together, holding tightness in their bodies, their shoulders up around their ears, their faces closed, they explained that there had been a family rift, which caused great pain and suffering. And they wanted to heal their part of that rift, recognizing they had no control over anyone else. They wanted to feel forgiveness for all parties, so they could move on. So, we had an energy session around forgiveness. And so much more.

I was aware they were clearing guilt from their part of the rift. Healing heartache from the pain. Releasing anger and resentment towards others and towards themselves. Reducing stress which compacts the spine and causes inflammation.

And finally, letting go of fear: the fear that they did something irreparable, the fear they were bad people, the fear they would be judged when they passed away, the fear this pain would never change.

When the session was complete, he looked twenty years younger and taller than when he came in my office. They both looked more confident, happier. They were at peace. I would say that was healing.

The physical pain and stress had compacted his spine so much, he'd initially had difficulty standing and walking. But after the session he walked freely, giving him physical ease of movement. Letting go of the emotional issues contributing to the situation gave him his youth back. His face looked younger, and he had more energy. Changing his mental beliefs from fear to acceptance gave him peace. You could see it in his eyes.

Just asking to be in a state of forgiveness helps heal the soul. He appeared more relaxed than when he came in my office. When we ask for healing, we never know how it will appear for us. We might think we know. We might think it should be obvious to everyone. "I want to walk again, easily!"

If this client had stated this for his session, it might have turned out differently. Certainly, the stress could have been released to facilitate greater ease of movement. But what about the mental and emotional components? Would they have healed also? How do you make sure you cover everything in healing? When we offer healing through being the hollow bone, we've learned to focus the session on whatever is for the client's **highest good and healing**—not knowing what that is but **allowing** it to be what it needs to be. Physically. Emotionally. Mentally. Spiritually. And letting Source Energy or the Divine decide what that is **without attaching** to what that is. And now we've come full circle. Again.

Being the hollow bone of healing brings the highest and best results, in the fastest time, without working harder because you aren't the one doing the work! Once you've stepped into this new way of "being," you'll never go back. Because, why would you?

I've put this all together with a guided meditation to help you open your heart, create your safety net with the highest and best, allow for the highest and best results, detach from the outcome, and experience healing. So, you can experience it for yourself. Because after all, when you become the hollow bone for yourself, you're in a better position to be the hollow bone for others.

Access your free healing meditation in
the supplement materials.

Register for your FREE Hollow Bone
Audios, Videos, Checklists
Supplement Materials
https://www.ask-the-angels.org/offers/vLUgb9ny

Already registered?
Access your account here
https://www.ask-the-angels.org/login

Next: In Part Two, learn how I 'stumbled upon' the originator of the phrase the hollow bone of healing after three years of searching, and how I opened my eyes to new levels of consciousness and healing.

PART TWO

The Originator of the Phrase
"Hollow Bone of Healing"

CHAPTER 8

What You Can Expect

When I first heard the phrase the hollow bone of healing from the angels, I intuitively knew what that meant. I understood it meant to be a conduit for Source. To be the pipeline through which everything came. But I'd never heard that reference before. And to be honest, when I checked on the internet, I couldn't find any reference for it anywhere.

But I kept looking. And sure enough, three years later, I found the originator of that term. And then I found even more.

I discovered that being the hollow bone of healing is a state of consciousness. When you tap into that state of being, you are tapping into the knowledge base of everyone who is also there or has been there. That's what consciousness is—a knowledge base of all. So, by tapping into the phrase hollow bone of healing I was actually tapping into the wisdom and knowledge of the ancestors who understood the term.

That gave my first backwards story even more credibility in my eyes. Because in order for me to discover the essential steps involved in being the hollow bone of healing, I had to tap into that level of consciousness for answers.

Which gave me chills.

"Learning to safely access layers of consciousness" (from my website) suddenly meant so much more than I had dreamed.

The Originator

Learn about Frank Fools Crow, the originator of the term the hollow bone of healing. Fools Crow was a revered Lakota Holy Man, healer, activist and mediator of those at Wounded Knee, and so much more. He shared about his healing with a trusted writer and gave instructions that none of his healing ways would be written about until after his death.

The Awareness of Harmony vs. The State of Love

Harmony is the word Fools Crow used for a state of being that embraces all life. Similar to the state of love that we begin each session with, Fools Crow used a prayer that embraced the unity of the world. Access a free guided journey that uses Fools Crow's method of becoming the hollow bone of healing, so you can be the hollow bone in the way of the ancestors.

Becoming vs. Merging

Fools Crow referred to "becoming" as a practice to become one with all things. To become "wiser" about everything. Compare this with The Healing Angel Protocol™ and *The Hollow Bone of Healing* where we teach the merge technique, a way of merging our energy entirely with our spiritual helpers. We become one and see through their eyes. In this chapter, access a free guided journey that takes you through "becoming" by using Fools Crow's method.

Visioning and Touching with the Eyes vs. Seeing with the Eyes of Love

Fools Crow talked at length about the importance of learning "to touch with eyes" (p. 61). In this, he was describing how his spirit helpers showed him how to see through their eyes. To see other possibilities for healing or curing.

In the Healing Angel Protocol™ and the hollow bone of healing, we teach that after we merge, we see through the eyes of love, hear with the ears of love, and speak with words of love.

Fools Crow shared that at first, when learning, we try to copy his words and be exact in what he was doing. Then eventually Spirit moves through us in ways that are unique for each of us, and our practices become ours. Which makes it even easier for us to apply being the hollow bone of healing to our holistic practices!

Healing vs. Curing

While it may seem like these are the similar terms for the same thing, they're not. Fools Crow found that everyone can be healed, but not everyone can be cured.

Find out the difference, and how Spirit is the one to decide the outcome.

CHAPTER 9

The Originator: Frank Fools Crow

I t took me three years from the time I wrote ***The Hollow Bone of Healing*** to when I finally found a reference to the shamanic phrase and its originator. I 'stumbled upon' a blog by Michael Drake from shamanicdrumming.com referencing Frank Fools Crow, "a revered Lakota Holy Man who taught that you must become like a hollow bone to be a great healer. He believed that to become a conduit for the source of all creation fulfills the destiny of the human spirit; to sustain the order of existence."

The blog also went onto list the four stages that Fools Crow used to become the hollow bone.

First, he called in Great Spirit to help him release anything in his way of being the hollow bone. Next, he saw himself as a clear channel, open and inviting. He felt the power as it came surging into him and knew that he needed to give it away. He understood that Great Spirit would continue to fill him with even more power that could also be given away.

I was so excited to finally find the origin of this way of being. Next, I looked on Amazon for more information on Fools Crow. I found a few books that had been published after his death on November 27, 1989 at the age of 99. In particular, I was drawn to ***Fools Crow: Wisdom and Power*** by Thomas E. Mails, who interviewed Fools Crow and received permission to write this powerful book after Fools Crow's death. It details how he did what he did and why he was considered to be one of the most powerful healers ever.

Mails asked Fools Crow why he entrusted him with this extraordinary information. Fools Crow indicated that the power we get through being the hollow bone needs to be given away. So does the knowledge of it. It does nothing if we try to hold onto it.

Nephew of Black Elk, Fools Crow was known for being the Sun Dance Intercessor, the Ceremonial Chief of the Teton Sioux, and a renown healer and medicine man. He was an activist who mediated between the U.S. Government and Indian activists at Wounded Knee in 1973 and pleaded before a congressional subcommittee for the return of the Black Hills to his people.

The more I read about Fools Crow and what he shared with Thomas Mails about his way of being the hollow bone, the more I saw parallels between what he did and what I've learned. Not everything of course, because I don't have his ceremonial and ancestral heritage. But there are enough similarities in the large concepts that I felt I had tapped into that level of consciousness, the hollow bone of healing consciousness, where I could access the knowledge and wisdom of those who had come before me.

Explore these parallels within the hollow bone of healing consciousness in the next chapter.

CHAPTER 10

The Awareness of Harmony vs. The State of Love

As a way of embracing all life, Frank Fools Crow offered a four-part prayer of thanksgiving. He used this for everything in daily life, for his rituals, healings, curings and at the end of each prayer session, thanking the ancestors for all they have taught us, thanking Great Spirit for his life and the opportunity to serve, thanking the descendants who will preserve these traditions in the future, and last, thanking all who were with him at that moment, and asking that they be blessed.

This prayer embraces the unity of the world, expanding the embrace of the whole of creation that includes the environment, our ancestors and descendants, and is the essence of harmony. Through embracing all of creation, the sense of brotherhood is amplified as a way of living.

In The Healing Angel Protocol™, when we are being the hollow bone, we offer the meditation of love. People report feelings of peace, just by that one meditation. They feel timeless, ageless, and weightless. They feel in harmony with all life. People use this meditation, not just at the beginning of healing sessions, but first thing in the morning, last thing at night, and many times in between.

I had no idea initially how or why this love meditation was such an important meditation, but seeing and understanding the parallels in consciousness between Fools Crow's prayer and the love meditation, I understand why tapping into this level of consciousness brings in similar feelings and experiences for people, even though our words are different. The vibrational intent is similar.

After offering his prayer, Fools Crow then asked to be the hollow bone for his clients, using the method I found in the blog.

Experience a healing journey using Fools Crow's method of being the hollow bone of healing. Allow yourself to be guided by this journey for your own healing or curing.

Register for your FREE Hollow Bone
Audios, Videos, Checklists
Supplement Materials
https://www.ask-the-angels.org/offers/vLUgb9ny

Already registered?
Access your account here
https://www.ask-the-angels.org/login

Next, learn more about how Fools Crow developed his relationship with the rest of creation.

CHAPTER 11

Becoming vs. Merging

When Mails asked Fools Crow if there was a way to focus his mind on his relationship with all of creation, Fools Crow answered, "Becoming."

For instance, when holding a rock, Fools Crow said he would talk to it like he would a person. And he let the rock talk to him. Telling him where it came from, and about all of its experiences. They become friends. And when finished, he felt wiser about not only the rock, but other things. His mind grew. He said that if the object was too large to hold in his hands, he would simply hold it in his heart. Great Spirit creates all life. And all things, whether they're trees, water, earth, animals, etc. have thoughts and feelings. All life can be learned from. He felt that the more he became one with everything, the wiser he became about everything.

In *The Hollow Bone of Healing: Miracles and Messages from the Quantum Field of Source Energy*, and in **The Healing Angel Protocol**™ where we become the hollow bone of healing, I teach the merge technique. This is a way we can merge our energy and consciousness with Source Energy, spiritual helpers or any aspect of the Divine. The way I teach it is to begin from that field of love using the meditation or your favorite way of being there, asking for the highest and best helper who appears on a wave of loving energy, knowing your helper is here for your highest and best, and then merging your energy entirely with that helper. My favorite way of merging is by holding the intention that our energy fields will merge so we are one. That I am seeing through the eyes of my helper. Gaining the knowledge and wisdom my helper holds. And being that energy for as long as possible.

After reading about Fools Crow "becoming," I taught an advanced group from The Healing Angel Protocol™. By advanced, I mean students that were confident in the merge, and used it frequently for themselves and on behalf of others. During that particular class, I mentioned Fools Crow and his "becoming" and invited them to "become" during the next meditation journey. We practiced on nature, using trees, rocks, plants, and so on. Everyone came back from that journey with eyes wide open, having new understanding and awareness they hadn't had before. One woman even said she'd felt nervous at first, but afterward was so glad she did this because it helped her to see the tree as a being, not an object.

Again, becoming and merging are just words. Yet because the meaning is the same and the intention is the same, the reverence for all life builds from them.

Access your free Becoming Meditation/Journey here.

**Register for your FREE Hollow Bone
Audios, Videos, Checklists
Supplement Materials**

https://www.ask-the-angels.org/offers/vLUgb9ny

**Already registered?
Access your account here**

https://www.ask-the-angels.org/login

Becoming and merging have more similarities.
Read on to learn about Fools Crow's visioning.

CHAPTER 12

Visioning and Touching with the Eyes vs. Seeing with the Eyes of Love

Fools Crow mentioned that when we're being the hollow bone, we are allowing Great Spirit to show us things through Spirit's eyes, sometimes with pictures, or new ideas of healing or curing, or sometimes ways to overcome obstacles. He called this visioning.

"By this, what would otherwise be impossible becomes possible," p. 63

(I found it interesting that my tagline for The Healing Angel Protocol™ is to make your unbelievable . . . believable. And that tagline was created before I read **Fools Crow: Wisdom and Power.**)

He mentioned that when we're being the hollow bone, we all are using our filters to do things a little differently. We each have our natural abilities and interact with Spirit differently. So even if people try to copy what Fools Crow was doing, eventually they would find their own way through Spirit to do what was required. When they experienced results, they didn't need to ask how it happened or if they did it right. They should just be happy with the results.

This is a perfect example of how to be a practitioner of the hollow bone of healing. When you are being the hollow bone, you can use either the Frank Fools Crow method or The Healing Angel Protocol™ (the hollow bone method). They're the same intention, from a slightly different communion with the Higher Powers. Accept what are the results, knowing they are for the highest and best. Hold gratitude for what is. Each practitioner may have slightly different interactions with Spirit and may see different results. And that's okay. Just be happy with the outcome, because Spirit is in charge.

This next part of the book really made me sit up. "I use my eyes to touch with gentleness and Love," p. 65.

Fools Crow mentioned that when visioning, he sees through the eyes of Great Spirit. In The Healing Angel Protocol™ we become the hollow bone and merge with our helpers; we see through their eyes. For example, when we merge with the Spirit of Love, we open our eyes to see with the eyes of love.

What that does is keep us immersed in the consciousness of our helper, or in the above case, the Spirit of Love. Being immersed in that consciousness helps us to extend that love with our eyes, touching the client or the object of our awareness. Love is what heals. Therefore, the eyes of love initiate the healing or curing, as it's coming from our Spirit Helpers. Touching with the eyes or seeing with the eyes of love hold the same intention.

> You might have noticed Fools Crow's
> reference to healing and curing.
> Read on to find out the difference.

CHAPTER 13

Healing vs Curing

In **The Healing Angel Protocol**™ as we become the hollow bone, we usually begin with all the same elements: getting into a field of love, asking for the highest and best helpers, knowing they'll bring the highest and best for the client, allowing that to be what it is, and detaching from the result. When we become the hollow bone, the helpers are different and unique for each client and presenting issue, and the results are unique for each person. Never have we addressed the difference between healing and curing.

According to Fools Crow, healing and curing are two different things. Anyone can be healed, but not everyone can be cured. Curing is what happens when the presenting issue is no longer present. A tumor disappears. The depression is lifted. The body is free from disease. And to cure, Fools Crow used a system of working with the person for four days, "touching then with his eyes," working with the Higher Powers who showed him how to make the impossible possible, working with herbs, tobacco, song, ceremony, gratitude to the helpers, and always touching with the eyes of love. He mentioned that through that love, they become deep healing allies with a rich friendship that continues through life.

Healing, on the other hand is coming into a deep sense of peace or "freedom from fear," p. 136.

Fears are debilitating. Fears get in our way. Fear makes us tense, and compresses our nervous system and our circulatory system, limiting our immune functions. Fear of death is common. Fear of painful death is another. So is the fear of being judged in the afterlife.

Then there are the mental fears. The fear of failure, fear of success, fear of not being good enough, fear of public ridicule, and the fear of being put to death for what you believe. In Fools Crow's healing, the opposite of fear is the deep sense of peace— the acceptance of what is, being okay with the transition from life to death.

He used a variety of tools to help the person get into his (Fools Crow's) mind. Then Fools Crow could talk better about the anger and pain blocking the person. When the person begins to realize that Wakan-Tanka is not taking their problems away, that death is a part of what happens in the world, then they can begin to move into additional tools for healing. Ceremony and song were his favorite. He would teach them the art of "becoming." Together they would explore nature, talk about the seasons, and relate this to life. Other tools included making 405 tobacco offerings to lay them by the altars. He also made a self-offering stick, teaching deep-breathing techniques, and provided flexibility for what each individual needed, based on the time that was left. And one of the last things he did was to tell the person to ask their family to sit with them as the person related all the healing that was done with Fools Crow, so as to review and re-live what had happened and help his client integrate this experience at a deeper level as well as help the family also have healing.

He agreed that many times when freedom from fear was present in a dying person, sometimes they live longer.

After reading that chapter on Freedom from Fear, I had a client. He was struggling with a lot of things. Having enough money, having a safe place to live, having a loving relationship, wanting to live his purpose and feeling that everything was holding him back.

As I stepped into being the hollow bone for the healing, I realized we were doing a healing, not a curing, for what was in his way was his fear. In his case, it wasn't so much a fear of death, as it was fear that he would die before he could do what he came here to do. I mentioned what I'd been reading about Fools Crow's work, and he instantly understood what I was saying.

"Yeah. That's it," he said.

His Spirit Helpers came in: the Spirit of Love, the Spirit of Light, the Spirit of Forgiveness, and Archangel Michael. I merged or became one with them. I saw them take him back a few centuries to when he first arrived on this planet, full of hope, filled with love, eager to experience life here, and to share his knowledge and wisdom. That lifetime ended up becoming one of control by others—and devastating for him. Moving forward on his personal timeline, I was shown that he then had chosen to cure the resentment from that lifetime of control in order to step higher on his path. And the way he chose was very mental, with no heart or love involved, but it offered him another possibility to come back so as to learn love. Each lifetime gave him another opportunity to add to his wholeness—until he arrived at this lifetime, where he chose to cure all karma, all deficits, and to use his lifetimes of learning to heal others. As each Helper assisted him, he cleared blocks to abundance, blocks to opening his heart, blocks to feeling good enough, and so many blocks! All in about twenty minutes.

The next day after his session, he reported, "I have a job offer, offering more than I ever dreamed possible. Plus, that will give me enough money to find a better place to live. And that will give me enough to be able to start doing the work I really want to do."

I am grateful to Fools Crow for this teaching! His ways of healing and curing are the ways of his ancestors, and much of what he shared has opened the doorway to more knowledge, information, and wisdom than I ever dreamed.

Ready to put this all together?
Ready to combine everything you've learned into your practice to help you serve more people, see better and faster results, and make a bigger impact on the world?

Read on for Part Three: Putting it all Together in Your Holistic Practice.

PART THREE

**Putting It All Together in
Your Holistic Practice**

CHAPTER 14

What You can Expect

I n this section, we put everything together, add in a few helpful ideas, and you have enough to get you started either building or expanding your holistic business so you can serve more people, see better and faster results without working harder, and make a bigger impact on the world.

The pre-session

Learn my **#1 Tool** to use before your client even shows up that will give you better and faster results.

The beginning of the client session

Check out the **Empowerment Strategy** that puts the client in the driver seat. Help them to be positive and empowered for their healing. Learn the most important question you can begin every session with.

The end of the client session

Find out how the **Mindset Strategy** helps clients feel supported on their healing path, to have a plan, and continue to be empowered in their healing, all of which fosters repeat, happy clients for life.

During the client session

Being the hollow bone of healing is absolutely the most important thing you can do to facilitate healing or curing. Even if you are adding this into your other work you do, you will begin to see better and faster results with your clients.

CHAPTER 15

The Pre-Session

S o, your client has made an appointment with you! You feel excited and maybe a bit nervous, kind of like the first day of school. (Remember that feeling?) Wondering if you're wearing the right thing. Does your hair look right? Do you have spinach in your teeth? Your stomach is in knots. Starting to feel concerned about doing this right and really making a difference for this person. Wondering how it's going to go. Curious if the client is open and friendly or fearful and closed. The mind is whirling with worry.

> My #1 Tool and THE most important thing you can
> do happens fifteen minutes before your client
> shows up and ensures you and your client will have
> the best session possible.

In this fifteen-minute timeframe, ask to be the hollow bone using whatever method works for you (Fools Crow Drumming or the method of opening the heart or your own way). It's okay if you need more than fifteen minutes for this. Allow the time you need.

What you are doing during this time is opening your heart and stating your intention to be the best hollow bone on behalf of your client.

Allow yourself to step into that state of everything and nothing. Where Spirit or Source does all the work. Where you are holding that state of love for miracles to happen.

Allow yourself to see with your mind, touch with the eyes, and decide with the heart.

Then, when you greet your client, you are touching them with your eyes of love, seeing the divine within them, being the hollow bone.

Access both the Heart Opening Meditation and Frank Fools Crow's Drumming directions for being the hollow bone of healing in your supplement materials. Use these recordings until you no longer need to rely on them.

Register for your FREE Hollow Bone Audios, Videos, Checklists Supplement Materials
https://www.ask-the-angels.org/offers/vLUgb9ny

Already registered? Access your account here
https://www.ask-the-angels.org/login

CHAPTER 16

The Beginning of the Session

The minute your client walks in the door, or appears on zoom, you are touching with your eyes, or seeing with the eyes of love. And you are empowering them to be in the driver seat of healing. They are in charge of their healing, but they don't know it. They get to decide if and when they heal or cure (along with Spirit and Source) and how fast and deep they want to go with it. I call this the **Empowerment Strategy**.

After greeting them and answering any initial questions they may have, here is the most important question you can ask them to put them in the driver's seat:

> How would you like your life to be different as a result of what we're about to do today?

Most clients are not ready to answer that question. They may have to think about it. You may have to help them rephrase their answer from all the things wrong with them to how would they like their life to be different. For instance, it's easy to walk in with a laundry list of 'my relationship isn't working, I don't have any money, I hate my job' and so on.

When you help them reframe their answer, you can ask them, what would your life look like if your relationship was working? Or if you did have money? Or a job you loved?

Really help them to get into what they desire. How it would feel to them. What could they do differently they can't now? Help them cultivate those feelings and desires around what they are choosing for themselves. Then they can manifest them faster.

Here's a simple checklist you can use to make sure you're empowering your client.

1. Describe how your session with them will work. Will they be lying down or sitting? On-camera or off? Will there be a recording? What exactly do you "do?" And what will your client "do"?

2. Talk about asking for the highest and best energies to come in and what that can mean. Letting them know that may include angels, guides, archangels, ascended masters, high consciousness spirits of love, light, compassion or whoever is for their highest and best. Help them to understand this is our safety net, so their results will also be for their highest and best.

3. Help your client understand that although they've stated a focus on how they'd like to have their life be different, we allow for the highest and best solutions. Whatever that may be. Explaining how healing can take many forms: physical, emotional, mental, spiritual. And while we assume we know what would be for our highest and best, we don't always. Help them understand the importance of detaching or "not holding on" to the outcome they desire.

4. Let your client know they don't have to repeat trauma to heal it. The angels say, "You've done this once. That's enough. Now let's let it go." Helping your client to understand it isn't more painful to let it go. It's liberating and enlightening. The angels and helpers do all the work. And if there's anything that needs to be understood from the past experience, the higher self will make sure that information is available, without having to repeat or relive anything.

5. Begin the session by bringing your client into a heart-opening meditation or visualization to help them release nervousness and pain and open their hearts. Remind them that you are empowering them to be their highest and best.

All of these steps together create empowerment and safety for the client. The client begins to understand that healing is not something that happens. It's something that *is allowed* if it's for the highest and best. If not this, then allow for something even better. Clients begin to feel that Source Energy is supporting them in loving ways. And they are so ready for their session!

The Empowerment Strategy helps the client to be their own highest and best healer for the session.

Need a printable checklist to help you empower your clients?
Access it in your supplement materials.

Register for your FREE Hollow Bone
Audios, Videos, Checklists
Supplement Materials
https://www.ask-the-angels.org/offers/vLUgb9ny

Already registered?
Access your account here
https://www.ask-the-angels.org/login

CHAPTER 17

The End of the Session

Coming out of a session is the next most important time for your client. What happens here is crucial for turning one-time clients into repeat happy, successful clients for life. There are a few steps to this strategy, and it's essential to do all of them to help continue to empower your client with a plan or strategy that supports them, and to let them know you've got their back.

I call this end of session **The Client Mindset Strategy**. You are helping them to frame their mindset for coming back and working with you, not because you are pushing them to "buy" your session, but because you will continue to empower them and educate them on the role of healing as they experience it, plus give them a plan for any future work together.

I find, especially with being the hollow bone of healing, that clients can be groggy after a session. The healing or curing deeply penetrates the layers for maximum healing in a short amount of time. And sometimes the brain has a hard time keeping up.

Therefore, the first step I do is **repeat the highlights of the session**. I let them know who their helper was, if there was a name offered. I share with them what messages or healing happened. I highlight how the healing connected to their focus and their highest and best, really focusing on the positive aspects of the session. This sharing helps the client to feel more confident with the session and integrate it faster.

With the second step, I say to them, "Now that you've had such good results with your session, **the next time we work together**, this is what we'll work on." And I give them an example of what might come up for healing.

For instance, let's say the client's focus was to release past trauma so they could experience new situations with confidence, and their session did help them release a past life experience that was limiting them now. I might then say, "Now you've seen how easy and effortless it is to release previous experiences without reliving them. And you're likely to find yourself in a situation soon that's new to you. As a result of our session you'll be apt to have more confidence to try it and see how it works for you. So, the next time we work together, we'll work on what else comes up when you are faced with new situations. You may uncover other layers of trauma that are ready to be released. Or you may want to explore new situations that you initiate, instead of waiting for them to come to you."

I then repeat, "So the next time we work together," and I add, "**—and you'll know when that is**—we'll work on uncovering additional trauma and/or exploring more situations with confidence."

The third step is that key phrase, "**And you'll know when that is** ..." because again you are empowering your client, letting them know that they'll know when it's time for another session with you. Now they have a plan. Not only that, they know you have their back. You have positioned yourself as the expert because you helped them to achieve results, and you can direct them where they need to go next. You have helped shape their mind-set into coming back.

These are the steps that turn one-time clients into repeat clients. You have laid the groundwork before the client arrives, empowered your client at the beginning of the session, and helped create a mindset of success at the end of the session. But what happens in the middle? What happens when the client is receiving their session?

Read on to discover the most important strategy
you can do to see more clients, have better,
faster results and make a bigger impact on the world.

CHAPTER 18

The Session

Being the hollow bone of healing can be a stand-alone process or an add-on to what you are currently offering. In my experience, as a stand-alone, the miracles and messages that transpire are so complete, you really don't need any other modality or therapy with it. Should you use the hollow bone of healing as a stand-alone process, here are the steps.

Before the session you've stepped into a state of love, where you are touching with your eyes, seeing with the eyes of the divine. At the beginning of the session, you greet your client while in a state of love that you maintain throughout the entire session.

You'll be answering questions about the session, and asking the most important question: How would you like your life to be different as a result of what we're about to do? You'll want to share more information on your safety net of highest and best. And you'll want to ask for their highest and best, without really knowing what that is, but knowing that's what we're looking for.

You'll be allowing the divine to do the work, helping the client to get into a heart-centered space for healing, and you'll be helping the client to feel empowered about the session and their healing.

During the session, you are everything and nothing. Everything because you are holding a state of love for the Divine or Source to come in and do the work. Nothing because there's nothing else for you to do. Just allow.

I mentioned previously that when our helpers come in, they don't always give their names. We may see them as a form. Or sense them as energy. Or hear voices. We may even ask them, "Who are you?"

If I don't recognize my helper, I may ask that question. And usually the answer is, "We would rather you recognize our essence, and not attach to a name." What that means is that a name can be limiting. A name forms an expectation for certain results. Having that expectation negates the Divine or Source doing all the work for the highest and best. For instance, if you knew it was Archangel Michael that appeared to help your client, you might immediately assume what is commonly thought about Archangel Michael—that he's here for protection, release of fear, able to fight off negative influences. Believing this could alter your ability to stay in the hollow bone and move you more into a thinking mode. And thinking with your head or relying on your experiences means you are no longer being the hollow bone with your heart. Therefore, some of the spiritual helpers would rather you sensed them with your heart, not your head.

I usually begin to narrate to the client what I'm seeing, sensing, hearing, knowing the Divine or Source doing. It can sound like a shamanic journey or a guided visualization. But the client is following along, experiencing it as I'm relating it. Or sometimes even before I say it, the client has already experienced what I'm sensing. I never know where the narrating is going. I am so in the zone of being the hollow bone I don't have an end result. I just let it come through my voice and allow.

Then there are times when there is nothing happening. I don't see anything. I don't hear anything. I don't sense anything.

I am an empty vessel. I let the clients know that when I'm quiet, it simply means I'm not receiving anything. Maybe, I tell them, this is their opportunity to be receiving. If so, I invite them to open their senses and allow what needs to come through directly to them and for them. I reassure them that it's not that something is wrong. It's more empowering for them to receive directly than through an intermediary, such as myself.

I have learned to trust that process. To believe that even when it feels like nothing is happening, **it's not that nothing is happening**. It just means that I am just not privy to it. Still, my students have struggled with this as well.

Here's an example of my student experiencing lots of helpers, but not aware that something else was happening.

> "Archangel Raphael was filling my client with loving energy, moving from the spiritual body to the emotional body to the physical body, and he was giving her healing to her heart and balance for her brain. Mother Mary was holding her inner child as Raphael was doing the clearing. Much of the healing was working on beliefs of unworthiness from this life and past lives. I sensed her ancestors helping and supporting her. Archangel Raphael strengthened her aura so any energy coming in would be filtered with love.

> "After the session, she wanted to rest more and not talk. But the next day, she felt at ease and felt a shift of positivity. And she mentioned having felt intense pain in her throat during the healing.

> "What I learned from this experience is that I should trust that the energy is what the client needs and just let it flow, let go of my fear and trust in Divine timing!

I was worried at first when she didn't want to talk, but then I realized she was integrating and needed time."

—Karen Sayago, Healing Angel Protocol™ Practitioner

Here's another example:

"I did not get the name of the spiritual helper, but felt it was the Angel of Love. I felt no energy movement or tingling but could see that the air sacs in his lungs were irritated. I felt moved to wave my hand over him in a circle and send Love. I shared with him that he is young and still has a strong life force. He is going to recover, but the Angels wanted to give him time to think about his actions. He is a heavy smoker. He blamed himself for the relationship breakdown. If he stopped the self-punishment, he would recover.

"I asked about how he was doing 72 hours after the treatment and was told he was still in the hospital. I did think he may not make it and questioned what I had told his mother about how he needed time to think.

"He was discharged from the hospital after 7 days. He had stopped smoking and is now breathing well, and his energy has returned.

"What I learned from this experience is that even if I feel nothing profound, healing can take place."

—Russell Sutton, Healing Angel Protocol™ Practitioner

You'll know when the session is complete. The energy sort of dissipates. Nothing more seems to be happening. You may even sense or get the message, "That's all we're going to do today."

When I know the session is complete, I tell the client to take a few minutes to integrate everything that just transpired. It's important to allow them to stay in that state of healing for as long as possible. Usually after several minutes, I gently bring them back into their body, where, like I said before, they may be groggy, or just kind of out of it.

At the end of the session I gently begin to highlight the important parts of the session, repeating them now that the client is more fully present. It helps them to remember everything, and to understand the session better. And it ties everything together when you say, "And the next time we work together, and you'll know when that is, here's what we're going to work on..."

If you don't know what you're likely to work on with your client, just ask your spiritual helper. They always know. And you'll receive that information in ways that make sense to you, whether you're hearing it, seeing imagery, sensing it or knowing it.

What I just described is an example of being the hollow bone without integrating it into your existing practice.

But sometimes we want to integrate it into what we do because we really love our modalities or therapies. We've worked hard to perfect them, to feel confident with them. We love them, and we love our clients. We'd like to offer our clients what we know how to "do," and there's nothing wrong with that.

> Being the hollow bone of healing can be an add-on to what you are currently offering.

When I first began to transition my clients from intuitive healing to being the hollow bone of healing, I described what it was like and let them know I was really excited about it. I felt that adding it would enhance our work together. I offered them ten minutes at the end of our regular session. By **adding it at the end of the session**, the client was more comfortable and relaxed and able to receive the benefits. And by offering it last, it became the first thing they remembered. As well as the results afterward.

Here's another way you can integrate the hollow bone of healing into your existing practice:

Follow the directions for Before the Session, The Beginning of the Session and The End of the Session and then you can use your current modality or therapy During the Session.

As a result of combining everything, you might experience subtle positive client changes happening without your intention.

Because love heals.

You might even notice clients rapidly having their unbelievable become believable.

Because love also manifests.

You might find your clients are more receptive to coming back. Again and again.

Here's an example of how integrating the hollow bone of healing into your existing practice can appear.

"We had been doing another modality, but I didn't feel the energy flowing. So I switched over to being the hollow bone. I didn't get a name of the spiritual helper but felt a very high vibration with tingles from head to toe. My client felt the same thing. That's when I shared with my client that because Angels work at the speed of light, this healing would not take long. That we were going for everyone's highest and best, as it involved a group of people who were not getting along. Within 24 hours, everyone was working together. Going above and beyond. They all felt a palpable shift and commented on how it must be a miracle.

"What I learned from this is that people highly value this work, and it can make your unbelievable happen at light speed. Angels rock and never underestimate the power of Love."

—Russell Sutton, Healing Angel Protocol™
Practitioner

Here's another integration into an existing practice.

"My client reported that she is struggling on every level.

"I would like it all to be better, and I'm not so sure about my meds". (Could not get her to be more specific.)

"I merged with Mother Mary.

"What I experienced using another modality were images and an inner knowing that revealed a "home' remarkable for its decay, a door within it (access or entry) that appeared progressively farther away and several cellular memory areas depicting a clown (Ronald McDonald) along with a palpable heat release.

"In being the hollow bone, I 'accessed' energy distortions in the time-space continuum as reflections of energetic disturbances.

"The thyroid was particularly highlighted. She was 'visited" by the energy of the tetrahedron and the icosahedron, and it struck me as odd that these are two consciousnesses would appear 'at odds' with each other to the linear mind. What was equally interesting was the flow associated with the icosahedron—way too fast! Her Sacred Panel was notable for aberrations in her emotional and mental bodies.

"My client fell asleep and was surprised at how 'quickly' the session went (it actually did not). She reported it to be peaceful and was relieved sufficiently that she decided to make an appt for the following week to continue. We discussed the significance of the images, but she refuted the notion about there being a problem with her home (she took it literally rather than spiritually) and enthusiastically reported that her parents were allowing her to live in their home for now. She found no association with the clown, however she confessed that she has been diagnosed with bipolar disorder. She did agree with the fast flow of the icosahedron being reminiscent of her mania.

"**What I learned**: It is becoming progressively easier to be the camera person in my client's life stories. Whereas I once felt that I had to 'do something' to effect change, this 'point and shoot' is highly liberating. It comes as a relief to know that any healing that takes place will do so in a time frame agreed upon by the client's Higher Self and Spirit. I am growing increasingly comfortable with trusting that something is indeed happening and that the outcome is what it should be. So comfortable in fact, that I must remember to make it a point to explain to patients about the shifts and integration of changes; some benefits are obvious, and some are not."

—Cynthia Higgins, MD, Healing Angel Protocol™ Practitioner and Team Leader

Don't be surprised when your clients begin to request the hollow bone of healing only! They'll love the results!

Here are other examples of practitioners being the hollow bone:

"My client wanted to clear old energy and be able to set clear boundaries with the will power to say no to others. She wanted better impulse control so as not to lose her current relationship.

"At the beginning of the session, I wasn't told who the spiritual helper was. I saw a red image of an eye with three purple curves above it, and below the eye was a green line that curved in three places to support the eye. I shared the image with my client. During the session, she received some clearing in the shoulders. I explained that the angels are helping to clear our past life trauma held in the shoulders, and that she was being given the gift of protection of boundaries.

"She felt much lighter after the session, and she had seen the same colors that were in the image that I had created in her session. Then in the days that followed she was able to successfully remove some people from her life that were not respecting her boundaries. However, we discovered that she was not quite ready to let go of one person in her life as she was still wanting to continue being friends with that person. So, in the meantime, she is trying to set clear boundaries with that person.

"I learned that while I am still unsure who does show up, I know that I can always ask for certain ones and know that they will be there along with whoever is there for the highest good and healing."

—Florence Buie, Healing Angel Protocol™ Practitioner and Team Leader

Here's an example of how sometimes we're guided to "do" something while being the hollow bone:

"My client was seeing me for her stomach ailments. I asked to merge with a higher energy for healing and messages. I just felt an immediate warmth. I put my hand on her stomach. I felt a rock like shape under my hand. It started to melt away and waves of healing energy were flowing from my hand. She reported much relief in her stomach. I got a message for her to go to the grocery store in the fruit and vegetables. Listen and pay attention to what sounded good to her and eat that."

—Janel Lemons, Healing Angel Protocol™ Practitioner

And:

"My client came to me with constant knee pain. She wanted to feel better. During the session, I don't know who came in to help. But all of a sudden, she put her knees down on the table. And kept them there the whole time. Something she couldn't do before without pain. I just watched. Every now and then her feet would light up, so I knew some clearing was going on. And at the end of the session, I got her some water and asked her how she was? She said amazing! She saw two large angels who were helping her knees. And after the session, she felt peaceful and without pain."

—Nancy Ard, Healing Angel Protocol™ Practitioner

More:

"My client was seeking to transmute anxiety and the energetic effects of her husband's verbal abuse; plus, she wanted assistance in grounding herself so she can move forward and announce her decision to divorce.

"The clearings seemed to emphasize her relationship with the Guides was REAL. She was shown past life perspectives that relieved her of the mental "why is this happening" tension and gave her Soul perspective on the "good" she was hoping to do for this man. Having a desire to remarry so as not to be alone, both of them agreed to marry. She saw "potential" in him. My client was offered the gift of "crafting" her consciousness and her future by way of contemplating her personal Truths about needs, boundaries, and as a result, clarifications for healthy ways to communicate ending the relationship. Post session she called to deepen her skills of grounding her nervous system and calm clarity about boundaries. She felt empowered."

——Donna Wolf, Healing Angel Protocol™ Practitioner

Plus, we can always be our best client!

"So, I've been suffering with sinus issues for years and this sinus infection this winter. I could not hear out of that ear. I called my doctor and said I needed to go in but could not because of the possible COVID infection. The symptoms sounded like COVID, so I was given the phone appointment for a few days out. I remembered while I was in bed, with my face hurting that we had just studied cellular healing in The Healing Angel Protocol™. And immediately I started working on my ear. Within a half hour I started to get some of the hearing back. The ear wasn't as plugged. By that next morning. I was totally clear. My ear was clear. There was no pain. No congestion. The ringing was gone, and I could hear, and this was prior to my phone appointment and prior to getting antibiotics. My ear's still doing fabulous.

"It usually takes a while before things start getting better. And sometimes I have to take two rounds of antibiotics. I've suffered with this since I was a child; it's somehow how my wiring is, and it makes it harder for me to breathe in. I just have a bunch of little problems with it. And this has been the first time that I've had some results without having medication like antibiotics or steroids coupled with antibiotics. So, I am on cloud nine right now. And I can't wait to continue working with it and hopefully eradicate more!"

—Janee Blackburn, Healing Angel Protocol™
Student

Just another nice session . . .

"My client stated a focus of clearing an old pattern of feeling undeserving and the pain associated with that pattern. She also desired to be a magnet for abundance (in the form) of money to assist in the successful remodel and build of a (spiritual) center."

"Serving as the hollow bone, I felt the energy and the words flowing freely, along with a sense of peace, calm, knowing and allowing. My client reported feeling an intense pressure of energy on the left side, and interpreted that as a clearing. She received lots of visuals for her center and was guided to get help from others."

—Dipti J. Shah, PharmD, Healing Angel Protocol™ Practitioner

Sometimes it's hard to trust your work when meeting resistance . . .

"My client wanted healing for her surgery, plus she focused on family and her highest good and community. So much came through! Archangels Michael and Raphael were there. The core of the message to her was about her heart. I felt the resistance when we were connecting to unconditional love. The angels led us through an exercise to open her heart. It felt like she needed encouragement to keep working on her path. She stayed in her brain space and used a lot of "I know" type of verbiage. She received the message that when she opens her heart, her community will show up. She was very resistance to the messages. After the session, the angels came back with a few more messages as she was integrating. She challenged the session and my security in what I was doing. The rebuff led me to question if I was in tune. But I stuck with it and stayed in my heart."

**—Grace Evergreen,
Healing Angel Protocol™ Practitioner and
Team Leader**

Learning to feel confident . . .

"My client came in for energy clearing. Mother Mary came in to assist with the heart chakra and other areas that needed clearing. I shared that I saw a beautiful bouquet of light pink roses. I smelled rose oil, and I saw light pink in the heart area. Mother Mary also worked on her palms and wrists to help her release the feeling of limitation. I encouraged the client to release old belief patterns that no longer served her. She cried and felt the release. And then she felt sleepy. I experienced more confidence with my communication in telling the client about the messages I was feeling and seeing."

**—Katrina Abeyta, Healing Angel Protocol™
Practitioner**

Becoming the hollow bone . . .

"My client felt imbalanced and had a headache. I merged with Archangel Ariel, the plant Cilantro, and the Spirit of Light. So much light came in. Her body felt weak, especially in the area of the solar plexus. The Spirit of Light brought in much healing. Archangel Ariel brought in love and compassion. My client fell asleep deeply. I had a clear connection and felt so much of her body. I visualized myself as a tube, or channel and allowed the spirit of Cilantro, the Spirit of Light, and Archangel Ariel to do the work. It was nice."

**—Marisa Martucci,
Healing Angel Protocol™ Practitioner and
Team Leader**

All kinds of helpers . . .

"My client wanted to release her headaches so she would have more productive time and not be plagued by them. The Spirit of Citrine, the Spirit of Tourmaline, The Spirit of Rose, and Archangel Metatron came in to help. I felt a body rush and chills. Citrine and Tourmaline came in as the form of the Star Tetrahedron. Citrine surrounded the client from the shoulders up to the 9th chakra. Tourmaline surrounded the client from the heart down to the feet. Rose covered her eyes and head. The energy of inspiration got stuck at the shoulders and again at the hips and knees, slowing the initial steps of manifestation. That caused energetic blockages that build in the head and cervix causing her headaches. Metatron says that the star tetrahedron will help with this flow of energy from idea to being fully manifested. I'm enjoying watching, listening and learning as the work is being done."

**—Marie Forrest, CHT, Healing Angel
Protocol™ Practitioner and
Team Leader in Training**

And . . .

"My client wanted clarity for her career focus and creative projects. During the session, I felt a presence, but did not get a name. I was sharing the messages of the underlying themes of not being heard, acknowledged, or appreciated in her life. The guides worked on her thyroid, hips, and heart to release cellular memory. As a result of the clearing, the messages came that she should stop waiting. She needs to shift from always supporting others first, as she thought that was her role. The client had tears in her eyes several times and felt the truth was being acknowledged as she released."

—Teri Ingle, Healing
Angel Protocol™ Practitioner
and Team Leader

To get started in being the hollow bone in your practice, here's a free 4-part training to assimilate the hollow bone of healing in the way that's right for you, helping you to serve more people, see better and faster results without working harder, and to make a bigger impact on the world.

Register for your FREE Hollow Bone Audios, Videos, Checklists Supplement Materials

https://www.ask-the-angels.org/offers/vLUgb9ny

Already registered? Access your account here

https://www.ask-the-angels.org/login

Being the hollow bone in your holistic practice doesn't really end there. At first, you may only think about being the hollow bone when you are working with clients. That's natural. What you're doing is building your spiritual muscle of unconditional love so that you are able to hold that frequency for longer and longer periods of time.

There will come a time when you find yourself with a friend, a family member, or even a stranger, and suddenly be in your heart, and experience the Divine or Source Energy coming through. This will help you discover just how incredible it is to live like this.

Find out how you can make this your daily experience,
and why you'd want to!

PART FOUR

**How to Be the Hollow Bone
as a Daily Experience**

CHAPTER 19

How to make this your Daily Experience (and why you'd want to!)

Once you make a commitment to be the hollow bone in your practice, you begin to notice how easy and effortless the sessions are. With more miraculous results. With very little effort on your part. Because you aren't doing the work.

You begin to see more repeat clients. More referrals. More clients aligned with your purpose. And your business grows.

What you are doing is building your spiritual muscle of unconditional love so you can stay in that space longer and longer. You are learning more refinements for what it's like to be the hollow bone, depending on what lessons you need. Each refinement teaches you how to go deeper into the process, trust the process and the results, trust the Divine or Source and yourself, and above all, allow the session to be for the client's and everyone's highest good and healing. To ask permission. To not 'push the agenda' for healing. To not assume everyone needs healing or curing.

I really feel this is just the tip of the iceberg in understanding how to be the hollow bone.

Because one additional important thing I've learned is that being the hollow bone has no invisible ceiling or limitations.

There are no built-in boundaries, such as "this works only under these conditions", "you can only use these hand positions", "you can't use this with cancer, but you can with heart disease", or "you need certain certification to do this". While yes, it's important to clarify what can and can't be accomplished in therapy, these examples of limitations indicate to me that the therapies are human-made, and dependent on human conditions.

In being the hollow bone, where the Divine or Source is doing all the work, there are no invisible ceilings or limitations because the Divine or Source doesn't have any. There is only Divine Perfection at work.

Therefore, there are no limits as to what we can learn about being the hollow bone or how we can apply it to our lives.

Because it's not just about doing this for our clients. It's about how do we live this? And what happens when we do?

Here's a perfect example:

I had the chance to really embody living the hollow bone recently and to step out and help people remember love. It was an unexpected event and I wasn't mentally unprepared for it which actually made it better, because my head wasn't in the way.

When I realized I needed to step up to the plate and be the leader, I simply turned it over to Source and said, "You're on. I'll just open my mouth, and you say the words."

And that's pretty much what happened.

Up until that time, I would sit in meditation for 5 to 10 minutes getting into my heart and having a checklist of what broad topics needed to be expressed before speaking.

But I didn't have that luxury this time.

This time, I wasn't "ready."

And yet I was.

It was the perfect place and time to step into a higher place in consciousness, and truly not even have an outline. It was the perfect place and time to be the hollow bone.

It happened naturally. It was easy, effortless. **I didn't work harder. I didn't have to 'work' at all. All I needed to do was BE the hollow bone.**

If I doubted how it would turn out, those feelings vanished quickly. The Divine was in charge. We created portals of Love and Light in the world. And we did this by embodying love and light.

After my initial "talk" and meditation, the profound sharing of results lasted longer than what came through me! People shared they were able to get into their hearts faster and easier. They went deeper than ever before. They had profound experiences. Such as:

> "I fell asleep, but it was more like I fell into a really deep trance. It was night and at the end of my day. I sat in my recliner while I listened to the recording and fell asleep. When I "came to" again, I got up, got ready for bed, then went to bed and slept for at least 10 hours.

> "Since then, it feels as though whatever happened while I slept is rather oozing into my days. It's calm. It's thoughts. It's patience. It's protection. It's connection, such DEEP connection . . . .to water, the earth, everything that is exploding in green and every other color, but especially green. And that's barely scratching the surface!!!

"There's so much more, but I don't have the words to explain the rest. I'm pretty sure I'm still processing."
TR

Here's another participant's experience:

"I've opened portals to everyplace inside of me connected with low vibration, like greed, fear, envy, guilt, laziness, anger. Wherever I connected with any other places with this kind of energy. Bring the pure, pure unconditional love for all oneness through portals into governments, religious buildings, in schools and universities, factories, internet violent video games or dark web servers. I'm so grateful for just being a pipeline to bring love in all those places." **MA**

(It was interesting to note that someone asked how this person had the permission to put portals in governments and religious buildings, and so forth. And the answer was, the permission came from spirit, not from a person.)

And another example:

"It's such a beautiful, beautiful loving meditation and I will share that I feel like I was part of everybody's meditation because I started also with my home and my husband who is struggling with the dramas of the current world. In my garden we have bees and then I started to back the love out to individual family members who have given me permission in the past and then backing up so far outside with looking at Mother Earth inside like this crystalline structure and then just surrounding it. It just kept getting bigger and bigger and bigger, not that I was forcing it on anybody but almost like a mist around those who needed it to soften the angers and the fears and the frustrations and the greed and just to allow the love to come through." **DM**

And another one:

"It's been a very powerful, cathartic experience for like the last 45 minutes. And I'm out here. I just moved, and I'm out here for the first time in the backyard standing on the grass, under a tree and just facing the sun. And when you talked about just imagining the presence of angels, I didn't see anything, but I had an overwhelming experience of being uplifted and having rapid body shaking. My breathing changed. I had many cycles of releasing and just vigorous shaking. And just that overwhelming feeling of being held and being nurtured and being supported at the highest level. And just really being in that very, very powerful space.

"Just being immersed in an amazing experience of being one with the universe and one with connection to everything around me. Being able to smell the trees and able to get a sense of the sun and the elements in connection to the earth and the warmth on my skin and my face. It was a very powerful healing and very powerful experience of unconditional love and being immersed in it. It was very, very powerful and I'm still in it. Just a lot of gratitude for this experience of really being immersed." **LM**

There were many more personal examples, and if you would like to experience this for yourself, the recording is part of our monthly Angel Healing Circle. This particular recording is called Creating Portals of Love and Light, and it's perfect for what to do when you don't know what to do! It's great for the environment. It's perfect for connecting to the Divine or Source Energy with love. It's super for feeling like you are making a difference in the world. And you are!

Because here's the thing. When you create from Love and Light, you are changing the frequency and energy of your creation to a higher consciousness level. When you create a course, for instance, you are creating a high consciousness course that helps teach others at that high level. When you create an email, you are creating a high consciousness email that resonates with those on that level. Not only do your creations resonate with those already on that level, but the Love and Light within uplift those who are ready for that consciousness and helps them step forward into it.

This is how you make a bigger impact on the world: by being in a higher state of consciousness, by living that higher state of consciousness, by offering it to the world in meaningful and guided ways.

This is why it's important to live and be the hollow bone. To impact as many people as possible in high consciousness ways. To help serve more people. To make a difference in the environment. To do what we came here to do.

To live love!

> Access the recording Creating Portals of Love and Light in your supplement materials.

**Register for your FREE Hollow Bone
Audios, Videos, Checklists
Supplement Materials**
https://www.ask-the-angels.org/offers/vLUgb9ny

**Already registered?
Access your account here**
https://www.ask-the-angels.org/login

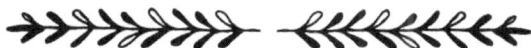

*To live love is the path of the shaman~
This is the path of the healer~
This is the path of ascension~*

This is the way home.

CHAPTER 20

Where to Go from Here

Being the hollow bone on a daily basis, doesn't necessarily mean you're going to be spontaneously giving a talk or seminar when you didn't plan it. Being the hollow bone will appear in so many ways as we are all unique beings.

For me, it's about deep listening--tapping profoundly into that voice of my soul that is so wise and loving and has all the answers. Following that direction and not trying to direct myself, even though it's second nature to do so. Trusting that what I'm "doing" is exactly what I'm supposed to be "doing", and that "doing" can be part of "being.".

Many times we imagine that "being" is sitting in lotus on a mountain top and meditating. But "being" really means living with intention and soul direction. "Being" means trusting in the higher power that's guiding us and following that guidance. "Being" means following that guidance even when it makes no sense. Especially when it's not what we "think" we should be "doing." "Being" means we feel soul aligned with our heart and our mission.

When we are "being" we are content. Possibly even happy. Peaceful. We attract more loving people into our lives. We attract more soul aligned people into our lives. People who are also "being." We are in harmony with all life everywhere. We are more consciously aware. Less judgmental. While we may not act in perfect ways, we are perfect in how we are "being" and what we are learning. It's a process. And it's a different process for everyone. It may take longer for some than others.

And that doesn't matter.

What matters is that you are on your path. What doesn't matter is how fast you go, because it's not a race. It's a journey. As there is no invisible ceiling, there is no destination.

You are never complete in your learning how to be the hollow bone. There is only the next consciousness level to access, and the next, and the next.

Which is thrilling to the soul, who loves to learn.

> In whatever way you might wish to incorporate living and being the hollow bone, I wish you well on your journey, for this is how we make a bigger impact on the world.

> May all Beings
> be touched with the Eyes of Love.

**Register for your FREE Hollow Bone
Audios, Videos, Checklists
Supplement Materials**
https://www.ask-the-angels.org/offers/vLUgb9ny

**Already registered?
Access your account here**
https://www.ask-the-angels.org/login

About the Author

When Phoenix isn't talking with angels, crystals and plants, she's writing and teaching. For the past twenty-five years, she has lived her passion as an intuitive healer and in 2019, created The Healing Angel Protocol™, 'the energy system that uplevels your life and holistic practice and makes your unbelievable . . . believable.'

Her career highlights include co-authoring with medium James Van Praagh, and being on stage with don Miguel Ruiz and his family at the Gathering of the Shamans in Sedona, AZ. Phoenix and her partner live on three acres in central Maine, and nurture gardens for beauty, food, and medicine.

Follow Phoenix on linktr.ee/phoenixrisingstar.

References

Drake, Michael. Blog: Shamanic Drumming. Talking Drum Publications. © 2001 - 2023

Mails, Thomas E. Fools Crow: Wisdom and Power. Pointer Oak/Tri S Foundation. 1991, Second Printing 2012.

If you enjoyed this book and feel guided to do so, will you please leave a review on Amazon or Goodreads so that others may also benefit from this work.

With gratitude,

Phoenix Rising Star

www.ingramcontent.com/pod-product-compliance
Lightning Source LLC
Chambersburg PA
CBHW022101020426
42335CB00012B/783